BARBARA DOREO

7 Day Health Challenge

Laugh Your Way To Fit

Contents

1

Introduction

What age were you when you remember being truly healthy?

Are you ready for this health challenge?

What do you need to prepare for this challenge?

Where will you shop for needed supplies?

Who will share your challenge with you?

How will you handle the stresses related to changing your daily habits?

How will you exclude people who might sabotage your potential success?

Get ready to appreciate your new self!

Ruthie was a happy, outgoing lady. She married Charlie; both were 21 years old. They loved ballroom dance and spent many Saturday nights at the Coconut Grove Dance Hall at the Boardwalk in Santa Cruz. They would swim around the Santa Cruz Pier after work several nights a week.

They had 2 children, 1 daughter and 1 son. Their middle class lifestyle afforded opportunities for extra curricular activities: ballet, folk dancing, music lessons, sporting activities, camping and more.

Through the years Ruthie gained weight, eventually she was wider than she was tall. Her disabilities multiplied as the years passed. Stiff joints, digestive problems, headaches, diabetes, heart arrhythmias, arthritis and depression.

The 2 children blissfully survived childhood, adolescence, the college years and became successful doctors. Grandchildren came along. Charlie was a heavy smoker and died of lung cancer at 67. Ruthie married the widower next door, Ed. They traveled on cruise ships due to Ruthie's disabilities related to her obesity. The cruises worked best for her because luggage handling, laundry services and meals were all included and provided by the staff on the ship.

Back home, one night Ruthie awakened with the need for a trip to the potty. On returning to bed she fell on the cold tile floor and couldn't get up. Husband Ed couldn't lift her so he gave her a pillow and blanket and left her on the floor.

The next morning neighbor Marion came to the door with fresh baked cranberry nut muffins. "Where's Ruthie?" Ed showed Marion where Ruthie was, laying on the bathroom floor. Ed explained what had happened. Marion was a retired bank manager, she knew what to do. Marion called 911. The ambulance came. Ruthie spent 5 days in the hospital.

Ruthie returned home with medications for high blood pressure, diuretic, high cholesterol, diabetes, arthritis, and pain medications.

Over the next 2 years Ruthie lost 100 pounds, she shrank down to 127 pounds. She didn't say a word to anyone about this. She drank more water, ate fewer snack foods, cookies, cakes, candy and colas. She ate more soups, broths and salads but she didn't give her delicious homemade chicken enchiladas.

Baggy clothes went to the Goodwill. No more struggling to get out of chairs and off of couches. She slept better. Aches and pains disappeared. Medications were not needed anymore.

At 85 years old Ruthie enjoyed life as she did in her twenties. Ruthie lived a full and happy life for another 10 years at 127 pounds and dancing!

2

The Reflection in the Mirror

Place mirrors in your home in strategic locations where you can watch your rolls of fat jiggle as you walk towards the mirror. Focus on that image. Is that what you want others to see? Join the Health Challenge and, like Ruthie, you can watch your body shrinking under those baggy clothes!

Just for fun you can photograph yourself in the mirror. Save it to share with your friends at the end of this journey. Loss of muscle tone and weight gain happens slowly as one birthday after another passes by. A busy lifestyle combined with pressures from work, bills coming daily in the mail, needy family members all take the focus off yourself. Thinking you can take care of your own needs after this present crisis settles down seems reasonable but another crisis pops up. There isn't time to recover from one to take care of yourself, the problems just keep coming. Almost everyone has this same problem. But, since there is no end to this vicious cycle, it's time to take control of your own needs. Don't let another day go by that you ignore your needs. As you develop the skills outlined here you will be thrilled about how you look and enjoy the extra energy you will have.

Look in the mirror again. Smile as a new you is coming now.

Diana J loved to sing and dance. She was very popular. Everyone loved her happy upbeat personality. She loved looking at pictures of herself and her friends. She admired herself in every window reflection. She always had a mirror in her purse to check her lipstick. She had no career goals emerging from high school but entered the workforce as a receptionist at the Ford Dealership in her hometown. She had a lot of fun. She partied, played, sang and danced. She maintained that position for 40 years. She had 3 children equally attractive and fun loving. Diana J ate what she liked, drank what she liked and may have indulged in smoking a bit. The Ford Dealership provided group health insurance which didn't teach healthful habits to their insured. Year by year Diana J kept putting off dealing with health issues. Of course they require self control and determination to make healthy choices. She kept postponing. She retired as the company remodeled their business plan. Her health went downhill quickly. Doctors gave her steroids to control her health problems. The dosages increased over the years and the number of medications increased as her fitness declined. She reached out but postponed the start of healthy lifestyle improvements until after The Holidays.

Sadly she passed before the planned improvements started. She is missed.

Let's learn from Diana J and get started on you now. Today is all there is.

3

Pantry Purge

Protein peps you up, carbs slow you down. Open the refrigerator, see what's inside. Are energy promoting foods filling the shelves? If not then purge the refrigerator of unhealthy edibles like sugar, syrup, breads and pastries. Keep the dark chocolate!

Neighbors, food banks, lots of places want your stuff. Keep track of the items that don't fit your new lifestyle. Make 2 lists, what you should buy and what you shouldn't buy. Great, you are off to a good start on your health and fitness program.

A chubby 60 year old named Carol A. said "I feel fat, what can I do?" She liked the ideas about changing her eating habits so she asked for more details. All this talking about how to eat lasted more than 30 minutes. At the end of the conversation she asked, "But what will I feed my husband and my son?"

Some unknown person in the corner said "All the crap you were going to throw out!" Carol was stunned. This was an "AHa" moment for Carol as she had complained that they were also out of shape. She got it.

Now attack your kitchen shelves and pantry. You know what you need to do. Pitch the carbohydrates, preservative laden cans, jars and cellophane packages. Make room for healthy foods. No preservatives, no "7 year shelf life Twinkies."

While you are at it, it's time to purge your bowels which could account for as much as 30 pounds of sh….. Follow this plan and you could feel light as a feather in 30 days.

Try this liquid diet for 5, 10, 20 or 30 days.

What do you have to lose? At the same time you can take these supplements daily for better results. Magnesium citrate, high doses of Vitamin C, Smooth Move herbal tea and lots of water.

Day 1-5 Veggie (celery, carrots, onions, cabbage, leaks, and all the green veggies) or Meat Broth (chicken, beef, turkey or fish). Make your own or purchase at the grocery store.
   Drink only half a cup per hour.

Day 5-10 Blend the veggies and broth into a thick soup. Consume only half a cup per hour.

Day 10-30 Eat the whole veggies and broth.
   Add Beneficial fruit from the list in Dr D'Adamos book
   Discontinue this plan if you have any problems and consult your holistic doctor for modifications to enhance your weight loss and fitness program.
   You can continue your weight loss maintenance diet by slowly adding healthy foods from your fat past.
   The pounds melt off your body much more slowly than they came

on.

Barbie's story. Barbie and her family were so excited to board a Princess 9 day cruise to Alaska from San Pedro CA. Once aboard they attended the orientation. Found all the exciting places that they would be visiting on the 9 day cruise. Pools, gym, library, game rooms, golf area, basketball, internet, music event locations. The whole family gathered for the 5:30 dinner seating. Louis, the waiter introduced himself and explained that all the food is available free of charge.

Each person can order multiple entrees, desserts and their delicious rolls with butter. Barbie did just that. She didn't have to choose just one meal, she had several with rolls and butter. Every night dessert included 2 servings of cheesecake with fresh fruit and chocolate sauce. Her clothes got tighter, she never felt hungry. Her stomach hurt, she had headaches. Finally the cruise was over.

At home she weighed herself. Nine pounds heavier in nine days! OMG!

Barbie is smart. She did what you would do. She started the liquid fast, took all her vitamins, exercised daily, maintained her high energy work style and lost those pesky 9 pounds in 10 days. She decided to continue the 30 day plan just to see what would happen. Success. She lost another 10 pounds. She felt great, no headache, bloating, constipation, no joint pain and her shoes fit better.

Clothes were comfortably loose. Life is good.

4

Shoes That Make You Move

Now that you feel like moving, get some comfortable shoes. Color doesn't matter but yellow gets me moving. Do you prefer RED?! Actually changing your shoes 4 times a day is the best advice to reduce strain in legs, muscles, bones and feet. The soul/sole of your shoe determines your posture. Try all the different shoes in your closet. Which ones relax your spine and call you to take a walk around the block?

Different styles of shoes use different muscles in your feet, legs, hips and low back. Changing your shoes through-out the day can help with pain and fatigue. Feet swell depending on your activities. Spending a long time standing can be tortuous to your feet and legs. Stretch your body out flat with your feet elevated. Turn on a fan to circulate room air and blood flow from your feet. Massage your feet and legs. Don't worry, you will be able to reach them more easily as you follow the steps outlined here in your new book.

Try on shoes with different sized toe boxes. Tight toe boxes lead to toenail pain. Is the shoe arch matching the placement and height of your arch? Does the heel slide up and down as you walk or run causing blisters that can become infected?

While you are out walking, explore restaurant menus looking for healthy dishes to satisfy your hunger and stay within the guidelines of your new diet.

Maybe your feet are the most important part of your body. Do you know someone who has lost their ability to walk? Being confined to a wheelchair for the rest of your life?

No. That's not for you. To prevent this from happening you can take steps now. Step by step learn to treat your feet to improve circulation and prevent foot neuropathy that plagues so many people. Treatments you can easily do at home start with a delicious comfortably warm water foot bath. Buy a foot bath bucket. Amazon has them for as little as $20. They are big enough for your toes to stretch out. Add a cup of Epsom Salts to the comfortably hot water. Add an Enaly 300AT ozone bubbler for even better outcomes. Soak your feet for 20-30 minutes. The ozone bubbler kills athlete's foot, nail fungus and improves blood circulation in your feet and legs.

5

The Dreaded Closet Purge

Purging unneeded things from your closet can make you feel young, light, fresh and happier. And why did all those things get stashed in the closet for so many years? You can take care of that problem right now.

People have different approaches to this seemingly overwhelming task. JJ said to take everything out of the closet and make a big pile on the floor in the center of the room. Then close your eyes and meditate on the vastness of the empty closet, visualizing the pure clean open space. Breathe. Feel the space. Observe the pile of clothing on the floor. Imagine which clothing items are ready to be invited back into the closet. Hmmmmmm. That might take a while.

Lauren's idea of the perfect purge is to throw out all the large clothes first. Large clothes need to GO! How else would she make progress losing weight? She can't enjoy dessert when it's possible that she would have nothing to wear to work tomorrow.

Jane had a seasonal approach. She said "Throw out all the clothes that don't match your latitude." She moved to Southern California where there is only one season, summer, from New York. She doesn't plan to go back to New York so she doesn't need those heavy fall and winter clothes taking up space in her closet.

Suzie agreed. She is moving to a warm Mexican climate and she doesn't need any heavy outfits. Purging to eliminate inappropriate clothing works for her and saves money in moving expenses.

Josie recommended throwing out the clothes with that little stain that no one would ever notice which is exactly what others do notice. She is so clever.

Linda eliminates the colored clothes that don't match anything else in the closet. It's the green color that compliments your complexion under the neon store lights but makes you look very dull in sunlight.

Judy said "Throw out all the clothes more than 2 years old." She loves to shop so this technique provides space for new fashions in smaller sizes to keep up with her ever slimming figure.

6

Intermittent Fasting Works

Everyone has their most favorite foods and least favorite ones. You will be surprised if you check out the Blood Type categories by Dr D'Adamo. <u>Eat Right For Your Blood Type.</u> You'll notice that many of your favorite foods are on the Highly Beneficial list for your blood type and many of the foods you refuse to eat are on the Foods to Avoid list

If you don't know your blood type you can order the kit and test yourself.

Refer to Eat Right For Your Type to make a list of Highly Beneficial foods that you like to eat on the left hand side of a sheet of paper. This will be your shopping list. On the right hand side of the same piece of paper write down the foods that you commonly eat from the Avoid list. This is your NEVER BUY AGAIN list. Make copies of this page and stuff one in your glove box, wallet, tape on the refrigerator, put them everywhere to remind yourself. Later you can look over the lists of Highly Beneficial foods for your blood type and add a few more tasty possibilities to your menu.

Stop eating sugar. Find new foods with more nutrition and fewer calories.

Growling stomachs are unpleasant. Distractions can postpone or even eliminate the craving to eat now. Brush and floss your teeth. Do 10 squats. By the way, if you reach down and pick up the cucumber that you dropped does it count as 1 squat?

The ketogenic diet with intermittent fasting has become the most successful food intake style recently to keep dieters on track for losing weight and keeping it off. The best part is that there are no packaged foods or powders to buy. The local grocery store carries all the products and ingredients needed. All varieties of ethnic flavors are available to offer variety; Asian, Indian, Moroccan, Mexican. Or no flavor, like the English! Reference Dr Jason Fung.

Lettuce wraps provide a wide array of filling possibilities, some fiber, and can be the go to for lunch, dinner and snacks. Deviled egg, beef, chicken, turkey, pork, fish and Krab, tofu and just veggies will fill the lettuce wrap for a delicious low carbohydrate meal.

Many types of lettuce can perk up an ordinary dinner salad. Watch out for high calorie creamy dressings. A tasty vinaigrette dressing is a better choice to reach the goal. And, watch out for hidden sugars. Read the labels.

Restaurant ordering can be easy and delicious and still maintain weight loss. Chef salad, lots of protein, no croutons please, with an oil vinaigrette dressing. No creamy high calorie diet busting dressings. Thanks.

Hamburger in lettuce wrap, grilled, not breaded chicken, beef and seafood. Butter and olive oil promote fat burning as long as no carbs are eaten. You will love this quick and easy delicious recipe that can be adapted to many taste buds.

Place a large skillet on the burner. Add olive oil and butter, a few spices like pepper, Italian seasoning, curry, chili, cumin or many other choices. Add chopped onion, garlic, all the veggies in your refrigerator, chopped. Mushrooms make a good addition and more garlic. When cooked to your satisfaction heap on a dinner plate, smother with hot marinara sauce, top with Parmesan cheese. Yummmy.

7

Move Your Bones

Stand, don't sit. Sit, don't lay. Burn more calories. Build muscle.

Exercise is a personal thing just like food choices. Some people are playing pickle ball in their 90's. Others are too fatigued to get off the couch in their 20's. Start your chosen exercise program slowly. Gym memberships aren't necessary. A half filled water jug makes a good weight for exercising. Start with light weights and a small number of repetitions. Move both arms and both legs. Move forward and back. Move side to side, rotate left to right swinging your arms.

Smile, it feels good to move. Try to exercise 3 times a day. A walk down the block and back in the morning gets the day off to an oxygen rich start. Bouncing on the rebounder mid-day for 2-5 minutes clears the cobwebs from your brain for a successful afternoon. Hula dancing with the wahinies on Youtube after dinner relaxes nerves and muscles for a restful sleep.

Exercise equipment runs the gamut from absolutely no expense to incredibly expensive. The same applies to monitoring gadgets.

If your living space is the size of a Princess cruise ship inside cabin you may want a gym membership close to home or work.

If health conditions or advancing age is a factor, monitoring devices will help you set the minimum and maximum levels of exertion. Technology is available to give you the necessary information to avoid stress, fatigue and worse. Stay within the listed parameters for healthy, beneficial results. Here are several examples: Do Smart Fitness tracker with 24/7 monitoring of heart rate, blood pressure, oxygen saturation among the higher rated technologies at $35-$40. LIVIKEY fitness tracker comes in all colors including purple for $20 with many features including Alexa built in.

Remember that all your daily activities can take a little more movement to improve today's fitness.

In the shower you can bounce in place while the hot water striking your back massages and stimulates blood flow. While waiting for your coffee to brew you can do kitchen corner lifts and push ups. A trip to the mail box allows you time to slap your opposite knee while you are walking briskly to improve your mental capacity and balance.

You can park at the furthest spot at the market for a little more exercise providing the weather is moderate. Don't do this in Death Valley when the temperature is 130 degrees.

"Exercise is medicine" -Author Unknown.

The need for particular medicines and their dosages may vary as your exercise program expands and your health monitors improve. Consult a holistic, alternative health professional, naturopathic doctor.

Susie was 12 years old when she noticed there were differences in family lifestyles among her friends that she frequently visited. Sleep overs were favorite activities among the young teenagers. She especially noticed the differences in eating habits and food choices related to the fitness of the families she visited. Susie started to incorporate some of these new discoveries into her lifestyle. Whereas her family required a heaping plate full of food to be consumed at each meal, other families used smaller dinner plates and served much smaller amounts of food. Susie's family was fat. Other families were lean.

Susie also noticed that she felt better if she prepared her own breakfast consisting of an egg cooked in a little butter. It tasted good, it filled her up and she wasn't hungry at 10:30 am. Many years later Susie is a slim, trim health professional. Think about it.

If a teenager can figure health and fitness out you can too.

8

You can do it!

Fitness equates to fun, flexibility and unlimited opportunities to participate in life. You can reach out to the limits of your willingness. Around the house you can tackle activities that would have been prohibitive when you were overweight, sore and tired. Changing the furniture arrangement is now a breeze. You can carry stacks of old magazines and papers to the trash in an instant and be done. No need to wait for a healthier person to help.

By the way, what's in the attic? Granddaughter Marlena outgrew her Barbie Doll collection of dolls, clothes, furniture and kitchen set. They may all be up there. Now you can go check on that. The basement has been an awesome storage area over the past how many years? There must be something of value down there. Today is the day for you to burn a few more calories looking for treasures.

Moving out to the garden, you can cultivate the dirt around those beautiful grapevines because your short handled trowel can now reach the soil as never before. Bending, reaching, twisting, leaning all improve your body flexibility. Keep moving. Repetition like pulling weeds is one sustained position that can lead to stiffness, sore muscles and joint pain. Every few minutes change your gardening activity. You don't have to do it all today. Save some gardening for tomorrow. Your joints will appreciate your wisdom. Moving the gardening tools to a safer place where they are convenient but also won't rust between gardening adventures is another activity that makes you healthier and fit. Off to the nursery to buy pansies and forget me knots to plant along the walkway. You can design an herb garden using pots that are sitting around the yard. Herbs will bloom into inspiring tasty healthful flavors. It's exciting to have the energy to plan, design and implement all these new projects.

In conclusion, wherever you live, urban or rural, whatever you do for work and play, and why you are considering becoming more fit, you are commended.

Lifelong good health will reward you in so many ways. Good health has a positive effect on your finances, on your peace of mind, on family and community relationships.

There will be time to tell more jokes, laugh with friends, go out and about and be able to take extraordinary care of yourself. Enjoy today!

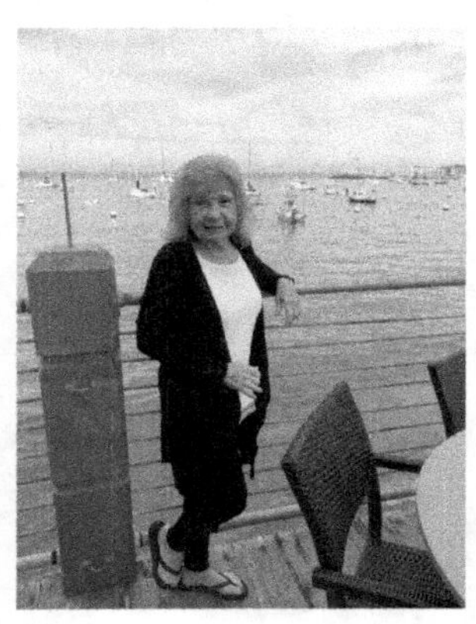

About the Author

Dr. Barbara Doreo is a Chiropractor and Dental Hygienist that has been helping people improve their health for many years! She is passionate about quick and easy ways to feel good and fuel your body. Her guidance has brought many people with many illnesses back to health and productivity - using many of the ideas in this book.